KETO
COOKBOOK

Appetizing Recipes for a Healthy Lifestyle and Weight Loss

JILL FOX

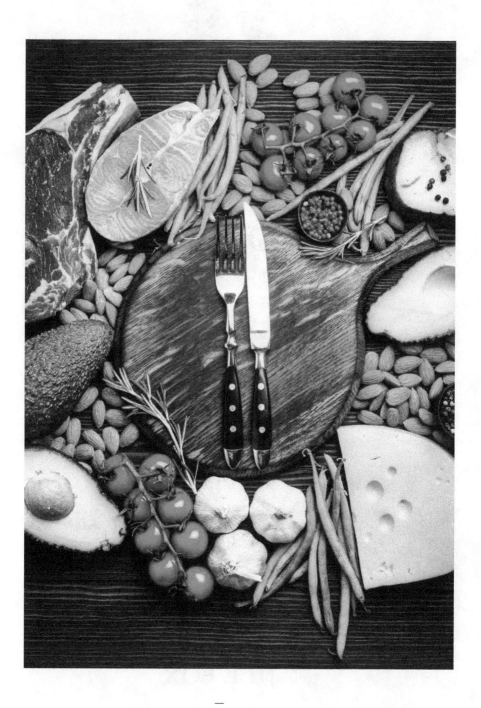

Table of Contents

Sommario

Introduction

The ketogenic diet, or keto diet, is a low carb, high-fat diet that gives many health benefits.

Many studies show that this sort of diet can assist you to reduce and improve your health.

Ketogenic diets may even have benefits against diabetes, cancer, epilepsy, and Alzheimer's disease.

What is a ketogenic diet?

The ketogenic diet is low carb, a high-fat diet that shares many similarities with the Atkins and low carb diets.

It involves drastically reducing carbohydrate intake and replacing it with fat. This reduction in carbs puts your body into a metabolic state called ketosis.

When this happens, your body becomes incredibly efficient at burning fat for energy. It also turns fat into ketones within the liver, which may supply energy for the brain

Ketogenic diets can cause significant reductions in blood glucose and insulin levels. This, alongside the increased ketones, has some health benefits.

Different types of ketogenic diets

There are several versions of the ketogenic diet, including:

The standard ketogenic diet (SKD): This is often a low carb, moderate protein, and high-fat diet. It typically contains 70% fat, 20% protein, and only 10% carbs (9Trusted Source).

The cyclical ketogenic diet (CKD): This diet involves periods of upper carb refeeds, like 5 ketogenic days followed by 2 high carb days.

The targeted ketogenic diet (TKD): This diet allows you to feature carbs around workouts.

High protein ketogenic diet: this is often almost like a typical ketogenic diet, but includes more protein. The ratio is usually 60% fat, 35% protein, and 5% carbs.

However, only the quality and high protein ketogenic diets are studied extensively. Cyclical or targeted ketogenic diets are more advanced methods and are primarily employed by bodybuilders or athletes.

What is ketosis?

Ketosis may be a metabolic state during which your body uses fat for fuel rather than carbs.
It occurs once you significantly reduce your consumption of carbohydrates, limiting your body's supply of glucose (sugar), which is that the main source of energy for the cells.
Following a ketogenic diet is that the best thanks to entering ketosis. Generally, this involves limiting carb consumption to around 20 to 50 grams per day and filling abreast of fats, like meat, fish, eggs, nuts, and healthy oils
It's also important to moderate your protein consumption, this is often because protein can be converted into glucose if consumed in high amounts, which can slow your transition into ketosis
Practicing intermittent fasting could also assist you to enter ketosis faster. There are many various sorts of intermittent fasting, but the foremost common method involves limiting food intake to around 8 hours per day and fasting for the remaining 16 hours

Blood, urine, and breath tests are available, which may help determine whether you've entered ketosis by measuring the number of ketones produced by your body.

Certain symptoms can also indicate that you've entered ketosis, including increased thirst, dry mouth, frequent urination, and decreased hunger or appetite

Ketogenic diets can help you lose weight

A ketogenic diet is also an effective solution for losing weight and decreasing risk factors for disease.

Research has shown that the ketogenic diet can be very effective for weight loss as a low-fat diet.

What's more, the diet is so rich that you can lose weight without needing to count calories or track your food intake.

An analysis of 13 studies revealed that following a low-carb ketogenic diet was slightly superior for long-term weight loss compared to a low-fat diet.

It also led to a reduction in diastolic blood pressure and triglyceride levels.

Other health benefits of keto

- The ketogenic diet originated as a method of treating neurological diseases such as epilepsy.
- Studies have now shown that this diet may have benefits for a wide variety of different health conditions:

- Heart disease. The ketogenic diet can help improve risk factors such as body fat, HDL (good) cholesterol levels, blood pressure, and blood sugar.

—
9

- Cancer. Diet is currently being explored as an adjunct treatment for cancer because it may help slow tumor growth.

- Alzheimer's disease. The keto diet may help reduce the symptoms of Alzheimer's disease and slow its progression.

- Epilepsy. Research has shown that the ketogenic diet can cause significant reductions in seizures in epileptic children.

- Parkinson's disease. Although more research is needed, one study found that the diet helped improve symptoms of Parkinson's disease.

- Polycystic ovary syndrome. The ketogenic diet may help reduce insulin levels, which may play a key role in polycystic ovary syndrome.

- Brain injury. Some research suggests that the diet may improve the outcomes of traumatic brain injuries.

However, keep in mind that research in many of these areas is far from conclusive.

Foods to avoid

Any food high in carbohydrates should be reduced.
Here is a list of foods that should be reduced or eliminated on a ketogenic diet:

sugary foods: soda, juice, smoothies, cake, ice cream, candy, etc.

grains or starches: wheat products, rice, pasta, cereals, etc.

fruits: all fruits, except small portions of berries such as strawberries

beans or legumes: peas, beans, lentils, chickpeas, etc.

root and tuber vegetables: potatoes, sweet potatoes, carrots, parsnips, etc.

low-fat or diet products: low-fat mayonnaise, salad dressings, and condiments

some condiments or sauces: barbecue sauce, honey mustard, teriyaki sauce, ketchup, etc.

unhealthy fats: processed vegetable oils, mayonnaise, etc.

alcohol: beer, wine, liquor, mixed drinks

sugar-free diet foods: sugar-free candy, syrups, puddings, sweeteners, desserts, etc.

Foods to eat

You should focus most of your meals on these foods:

meat: red meat, steak, ham, sausage, bacon, chicken, and turkey

fatty fish: salmon, trout, tuna, and mackerel

eggs: whole pastured eggs or omega-3s

butter and cream: grass-fed butter and heavy cream

cheese: non-processed cheeses such as cheddar, goat, cream, blue, or mozzarella cheese

nuts and seeds: almonds, walnuts, flaxseeds, pumpkin seeds, chia seeds, etc.

healthy oils: extra virgin olive oil, coconut oil, and avocado oil

avocado: whole avocado or freshly made guacamole

low carb vegetables: green vegetables, tomatoes, onions, peppers, etc.

seasonings: salt, pepper, herbs, and spices

It's best to base your diet primarily on whole, single-ingredient foods. Here's a list of 44 healthy low-carb foods.

Healthy keto snacks

In case you get the urge to eat between meals, here are some healthy, keto-approved snacks:

fatty meat or fish
cheese
a handful of nuts or seeds
keto sushi bites
olives
one or two hard-boiled or deviled eggs
keto-friendly snack bars
90 percent dark chocolate
whole Greek yogurt mixed with nut butter and cocoa powder
peppers and guacamole
strawberries and plain cottage cheese
celery with salsa and guacamole
beef jerky
smaller portions of leftover meals
fat bombs

Keto tips and tricks

Although starting the ketogenic diet can be difficult, there are several tips and tricks you can use to make it easier.

Start by familiarizing yourself with food labels and checking the grams of fat, carbohydrates, and fiber to determine how your favorite foods can fit into your diet.
Planning your meals can also be beneficial and can help you save extra time during the week.

Tips for eating out on a ketogenic diet

Many restaurant meals can be made keto-friendly.
Most restaurants offer some type of meat or fish dish. Order this food and replace any high-carb food with extra vegetables.
Egg meals are also a good option, such as an omelet or eggs and bacon.
Another favorite meal is burgers without a bun. You could also replace the fries with veggies. Add extra avocado, cheese, bacon, or eggs.
In Mexican restaurants, you can enjoy any type of meat with extra cheese, guacamole, salsa, and sour cream.
For dessert, ask for a tray of mixed cheeses or berries with cream.

At least, in the beginning, it's crucial to eat until you're full and avoid cutting calories too much. Usually, a ketogenic diet involves weight loss without intentional calorie restriction.

In this Keto cookbook, you can organize your Keto diet with the different dishes you'll find for meals throughout the day. Enjoy!

Breakfast

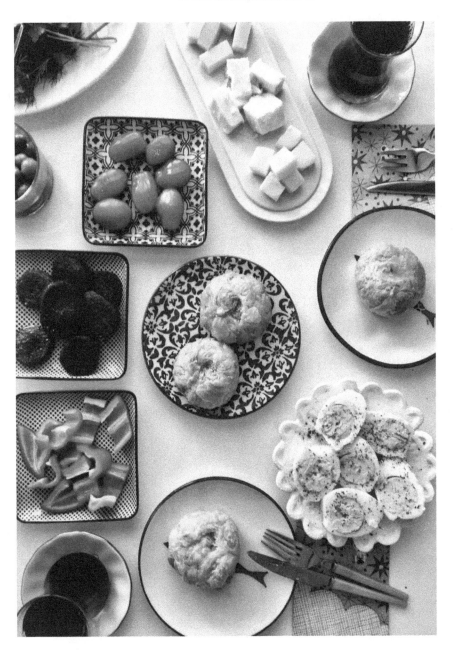

Fried Apple Slices

Preparation time: 10 minutes
Cooking time: 6 hours
Servings: 6

Ingredients:
1 teaspoon ground cinnamon
3 tablespoons cornstarch
3 pounds Granny Smith apples
¼ teaspoon nutmeg, freshly grated
cup sugar, granulated
tablespoons butter

Directions:
Put the apple slices in the crock pot and stir in nutmeg, cinnamon, sugar and cornstarch.
Top with butter and cover the lid.
Cook on LOW for about 6 hours, stirring about halfway.
Dish out to serve hot.

Nutrition
Calories: 234
Fat: 4.1g
Carbohydrates: 52.7g

Pumpkin pie with sorghum

Preparation time: 10 minutes
Cooking time: 8 hours
Servings: 4

Ingredients:
Pumpkin pie spice-1 tbsp.
Maple syrup-2 tbsp. s.
Vanilla extract-1 tsp.
Almond milk (unsweetened) - 1 cup
Sorghum-1 cup
Pumpkin puree-3/4 cup

Directions:
In a slow cooker combine all the above ingredients and mix well.
Add two cups of water to it and mix again.
Let the mixture cook for 8 hours so that the sorghum gets tender and the liquid gets dissolved.
Serve hot.

Nutrition:
Calories: 221,
Total fat: 3g,
Cholesterol: 0mg,
Sodium: 52 mg,
Carbohydrate: 27g,
Dietary fiber: 5g, Protein: 6g

Veggie Hash Brown Mix

Preparation time: 10 minutes
Cooking time: 6 hours and 5 minutes
Servings: 2

Ingredients:
1 tablespoon olive oil
½ cup white mushrooms, chopped
½ yellow onion, chopped
¼ teaspoon garlic powder ¼ teaspoon onion powder
¼ cup sour cream
10 ounces hash browns
¼ cup cheddar cheese, shredded
Salt and black pepper to the taste ½ tablespoon parsley, chopped

Directions:
Heat up a pan with the oil over medium heat, add the onion and mushrooms, stir and cook for 5 minutes.
Transfer this to the slow cooker, add hash browns and the other ingredients, toss, put the lid on and cook on Low for 6 hours.
Divide between plates and for breakfast.
Nutrition:

Calories 571,
Fat 35.6,
Fiber 5.4,
Carbs 54.9, Protein 9.7

Apple with Chia Mix

Preparation time: 10 minutes
Cooking time: 8 hours
Servings: 2

Ingredients:
¼ cup chia seeds
2 apples, cored and roughly cubed
cup almond milk
tablespoons maple syrup
1 teaspoon vanilla extract
½ tablespoon cinnamon powder
Cooking spray

Directions:
Grease your slow cooker with the cooking spray, add the chia seeds, milk and the other ingredients, toss, put the lid on and cook on Low for 8 hours. Divide the mix into bowls and serve for breakfast.

Nutrition:
Calories 453,
Fat 29.3,
Fiber 8,
Carbs 51.1, Protein 3.4

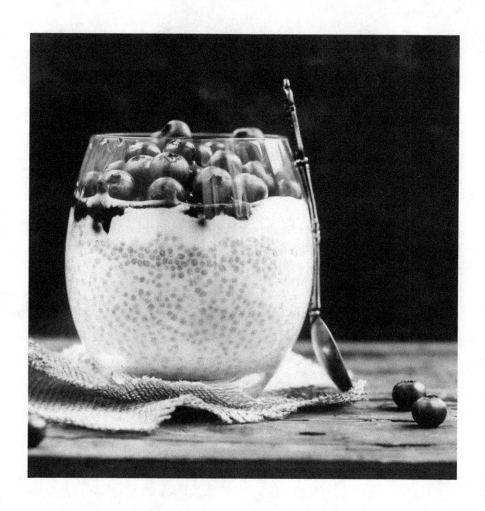

Green Vegetable Quiche

Preparation Time: 20 minutes
Cooking Time: 20 minutes
Servings: 4

Ingredients:
6 organic eggs
1/2 cup unsweetened almond milk
Salt and ground black pepper, as required
2 cups fresh baby spinach, chopped
1/2 cup green bell pepper, seeded and chopped
1 scallion, chopped
1/4 cup fresh cilantro, chopped
1 tablespoon fresh chives, minced
3 tablespoons mozzarella cheese, grated

Directions:
Preheat your oven to 400°F. Lightly grease a pie dish. In a bowl, add eggs, almond milk, salt, and black pepper, and beat until well combined. Set aside. In another bowl, add the vegetables and herbs and mix well. At the bottom of the prepared pie dish, place the veggie mixture evenly and top with the egg mixture. Let the quiche bake for about 20 minutes. Remove the pie dish from the oven and immediately sprinkle with the Parmesan cheese. Set aside for about 5 minutes before slicing. Cut into desired sized wedges and serve warm.

Nutrition:
Calories: 298
Fat: 10.4g
Fiber: 5.9g
 Carbohydrates: 4.1 g
Protein: 7.9g

21

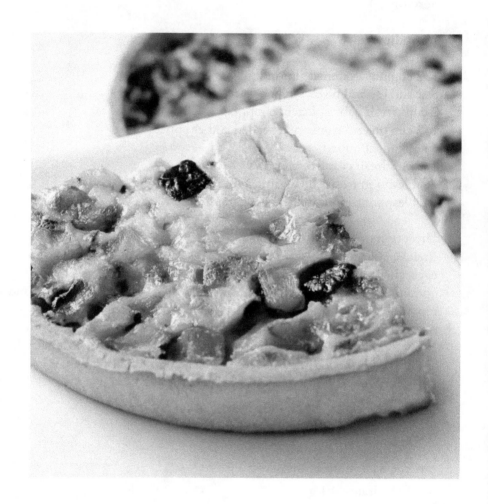

Sausage and Potato Mix

Preparation time: 10 minutes
Cooking time: 6 hours
Servings: 2

Ingredients:
2 sweet potatoes, peeled and roughly cubed
1 green bell pepper, minced
½ yellow onion, chopped
4 ounces smoked Andouille sausage, sliced
1 cup cheddar cheese, shredded
¼ cup Greek yogurt
¼ teaspoon basil, dried
1 cup chicken stock
Salt and black pepper to the taste
1 tablespoon parsley, chopped

Directions:
In your slow cooker, combine the potatoes with the bell pepper, sausage and the other ingredients, toss, put the lid on and cook on Low for 6 hours.
Divide between plates and serve for breakfast.

Nutrition:
Calories 623,
Fat 35.7,
Fiber 7.6,
Carbs 53.1,
Protein 24.8

Chicken

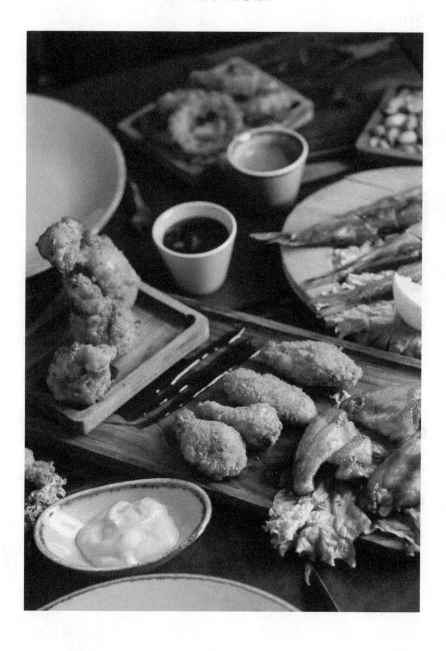

Chicken Spinach Salad

Preparation Time: 15 minutes
Cooking Time: 0 minutes
Servings: 3

Ingredients:
2 1/2 cups of spinach
4 1/2 ounces of boiled chicken
boiled eggs
1/2 cup of chopped cucumber
slices of bacon
1 small avocado
1 tablespoon olive oil
1/2 teaspoon of coconut oil
Pinch of Salt
Pepper

Directions:
Dice the boiled eggs.
Slice boiled chicken, bacon, avocado, spinach, cucumber, and combine them in a bowl. Then add diced boiled eggs.
Drizzle with some oil. Mix well.
Add salt and pepper to taste.
Enjoy.

Nutrition:
Calories: 265
Fat: 9.5g
Fiber: 10.5g
Carbohydrates:3.3 g
Protein: 14.1 g

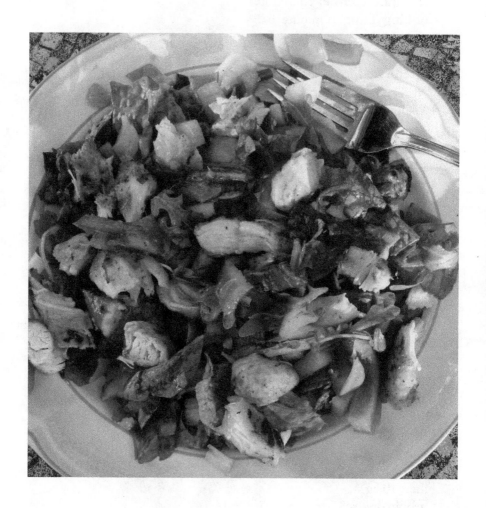

Chicken Thigh and Kale Stew

Preparation time: 20 minutes
Cooking time: 6 hours
Servings: 6

Ingredients:
3 tablespoons extra-virgin olive oil, divided
pound (454 g) boneless chicken thighs, diced into 1½-inch pieces
½ sweet onion, chopped
teaspoons minced garlic
2 cups chicken broth
2 celery stalks, diced
1 carrot, diced
1 teaspoon dried thyme
1 cup shredded kale
1 cup coconut cream
Salt, for seasoning
Freshly ground black pepper, for seasoning

Directions:
Lightly grease the insert of the slow cooker with 1 tablespoon of the olive oil.
In a large skillet over medium-high heat, heat the remaining 2 tablespoons of the olive oil. Add the chicken and sauté until it is just cooked through, about 7 minutes.
Add the onion and garlic and sauté for an additional 3 minutes.
Transfer the chicken mixture to the insert, and stir in the broth, celery, carrot, and thyme.
Cover and cook on low for 6 hours.
Stir in the kale and coconut cream.
Season with salt and pepper, and serve warm.

Nutrition:
calories: 277 | fat: 22.0g | protein: 17.0g | carbs: 6.0g | net carbs: 4.0g | fiber: 2.0g

27

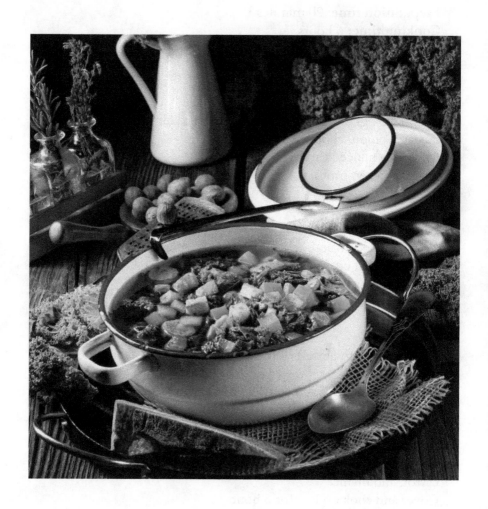

Thai Chicken Salad Bowl

Preparation Time: 12 minutes
Cooking Time: 15 minutes
Servings: 2

Ingredients:
Marinade:
1 clove garlic, minced
1 tbsp. grated ginger
small red chili, finely chopped
1/2 stalk lemongrass, finely chopped
tbsp. fresh lime juice
1 tsp. fish sauce 1 tbsp. coconut aminos Salad:
8 oz (226g) (2-pieces) chicken breasts
1/2 cup shredded red cabbage
1/2 cup shredded green cabbage
2/3 cup grated carrot
1 tbsp. chopped mint
1/2 cup chopped cilantro
1 tbsp. chopped chives 1/4 cup blanched almonds
Dressing:
3 tbsp. extra virgin olive oil
Salt and pepper, to taste

Directions:
Oven: 400 F
Combine the garlic, ginger, red chili, lemongrass, lime juice, fish sauce, and coconut aminos in a bowl for marinating and crush with a mortar. Flatten the chicken breasts with a meat mallet. Add the chicken in a bowl and add half of the marinade, and coat the chicken evenly. Make it cool in the refrigerator for a maximum of 30 minutes or an hour. Combine both cabbages, carrot, mint, cilantro, and chives in a bowl. In a baking tray, spread out the almonds and roast in the oven for 5-8 minutes, set aside. Grill the chicken in a griddle. Cook through then slice. Mix int the remaining ingredients.
Nutrition: Calories: 351; Fat: 15.7g; Fiber: 11.4g; Carbohydrates:3.1 g Protein: 12.5g

---

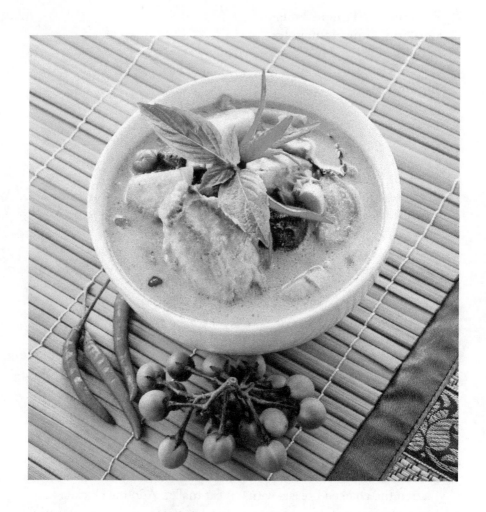

Double-Cheese Ranch Chicken

Preparation time: 15 minutes
Cookings time: 20 minutes
Servings: 4

Ingredients:
2 chicken breasts
2 tablespoons butter, melted
1 teaspoon salt
½ teaspoon garlic powder
½ teaspoon cayenne pepper
½ teaspoon black peppercorns, crushed
½ tablespoon ranch seasoning mix
4 ounces (113 g) Ricotta cheese, room temperature
½ cup Monterey-Jack cheese, grated
4 slices bacon, chopped
¼ cup scallions, chopped

Directions:
Start by preheating your oven to 370°F (188°C).
Drizzle the chicken with melted butter. Rub the chicken with salt, garlic
powder, cayenne pepper, black pepper, and ranch seasoning mix.
Heat a cast iron skillet over medium heat. Cook the chicken for 3 to 5 minutes
per side. Transfer the chicken to a lightly greased baking dish.
Add cheese and bacon. Bake about 12 minutes. Top with scallions just before
serving. Bon appétit!

Nutrition:
calories: 290
fat: 19.3g
protein: 25.1g
carbs: 2.5g
net carbs: 2.5g
fiber: 0g

Salsa Turkey Cutlet and Zucchini Stir-Fry

Preparation time: 10 minutes
Cooking time: 15 minutes
Servings: 4

Ingredients:
2 tablespoons olive oil
1 pound (454 g) turkey cutlets
red onion, sliced
garlic cloves, minced
1 chili pepper, chopped
Sea salt and ground black pepper, to taste
½ teaspoon cayenne pepper
½ teaspoon dried basil
1 teaspoon dried rosemary
½ teaspoon cumin seeds
½ teaspoon mustard seeds
1 zucchini, spiralized
½ cup salsa

Directions:
Heat 1 tablespoon of the olive oil in a frying pan over a moderate
flame. Cook the turkey cutlets until they are golden brown or about 10
minutes; shred the meat with two forks and reserve.
Heat the remaining tablespoon of olive oil in the same frying pan.
Now, sauté the onion, garlic, and chili pepper until they have softened.
Add the spices and stir in the reserved turkey. Fold in the zucchini and
cook for 3 minutes or until it is tender and everything is cooked
through. Serve with salsa on the side. Enjoy!

Nutrition:
calories: 211 | fat: 9.1g | protein: 26.1g | carbs: 5.5g | net carbs: 4.4g |
fiber: 1.1g

Turkey and Canadian Bacon Pizza

Preparation time: 10 minutes
Cooking time: 32 minutes
Servings: 4

Ingredients:
½ pound (227 g) ground turkey
½ cup Parmesan cheese, freshly grated
½ cup Mozzarella cheese, grated
Salt and ground black pepper, to taste
bell pepper, sliced
slices Canadian bacon, chopped
1 tomato, chopped
1 teaspoon oregano
½ teaspoon basil

Directions:
In mixing bowl, thoroughly combine the ground turkey, cheese, salt, and black pepper.
Then, press the cheese-chicken mixture into a parchment-lined baking pan.
Bake in the preheated oven, at 390°F (199°C) for 22 minutes.
Add bell pepper, bacon, tomato, oregano, and basil. Bake an additional 10 minutes and serve warm. Bon appétit!

Nutrition:
calories: 361
fat: 22.6g
protein: 32.5g
carbs: 5.8g
net carbs: 5.2g
fiber: 0.6g

Pork

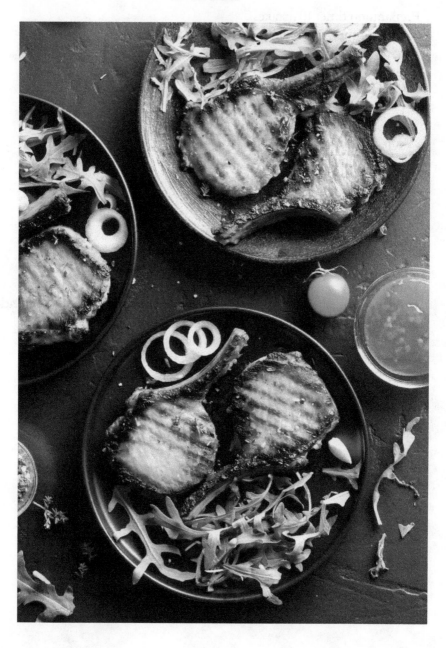

Beef Wellington

Preparation Time: 20 minutes
Cooking Time: 40 minutes
Servings: 4

Ingredients:
2 (4-ounce) grass-fed beef tenderloin steaks, halved
Salt and ground black pepper, as required
1 tablespoon butter
1 cup mozzarella cheese, shredded
1/2 cup almond flour
4 tablespoons liver pate

Directions:
Preheat your oven to 400°F. Grease a baking sheet. Season the steaks with pepper and salt. Sear the beef steaks for about 2–3 minutes per side. In a microwave-safe bowl, add the mozzarella cheese and microwave for about 1 minute. Remove from the microwave and stir in the almond flour until a dough forms. Place the dough between 2 parchment paper pieces and, with a rolling pin, roll to flatten it. Remove the upper parchment paper piece. Divide the rolled dough into four pieces. Place one tablespoon of pate onto each dough piece and top with one steak piece. Cover each steak piece with dough completely. Arrange the covered steak pieces onto the prepared baking sheet in a single layer.
Baking time: 20-30 minutes
Serve warm.

Nutrition:
Calories: 412
Fat: 15.6g
Fiber: 9.1g
Carbohydrates:4.9 g
Protein: 18.5g

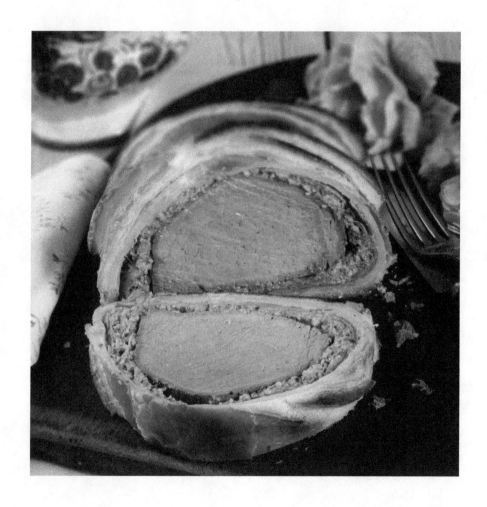

Texas Pulled Boston Butt

Preparation time: 15 minutes
Cooking time: 3 hours
Servings: 4

Ingredients:
Kosher salt, to season
1 teaspoon paprika
½ teaspoon oregano
½ teaspoon rosemary
1 teaspoon mustard seeds
½ teaspoon chipotle powder
1 teaspoon black peppercorns, whole
3 tablespoons apple cider vinegar
1 cup tomato sauce
1½ pounds (680 g) Boston butt

Directions:
Thoroughly combine all ingredients, except for the Boston butt, in a big casserole dish. Now, place Boston butt on top skin-side up.
Bake in the preheated oven at 300°F (150°C) for about 3 hours, checking and turning every 30 minutes.
Cut the skin off and shred the pork with two forks; discard any fatty bits.
Serve with coleslaw and the bowl of cooking juices on the side for dipping. Bon appétit!

Nutrition:
calories: 340 | fat: 21.1g | protein: 30.7g | carbs: 4.3g | net carbs: 3.2g | fiber: 1.1g

Creamy Dijon Pork Filet Mignon

Preparation time: 10 minutes
Cooking time: 10 minutes
Servings: 6

Ingredients:
2 teaspoons lard, at room temperature
2 pounds (907 g) pork filet mignon, cut into bite-sized chunks
Flaky salt and ground black pepper, to season
1 tablespoon Dijon mustard
1 cup double cream

Directions:
Melt the lard in a saucepan over moderate heat; now, sear the filet mignon for 2 to 3 minutes per side. Season with salt and pepper to taste.
Fold in the Dijon mustard and cream. Reduce the heat to medium-low and continue to cook for a further 6 minutes or until the sauce has reduced slightly.
Serve in individual plates, garnished with cauli rice if desired. Enjoy!

Nutrition:
calories: 302
fat: 16.5g
protein: 34.1g
carbs: 2.2g
net carbs: 2.1g
fiber: 0.1g

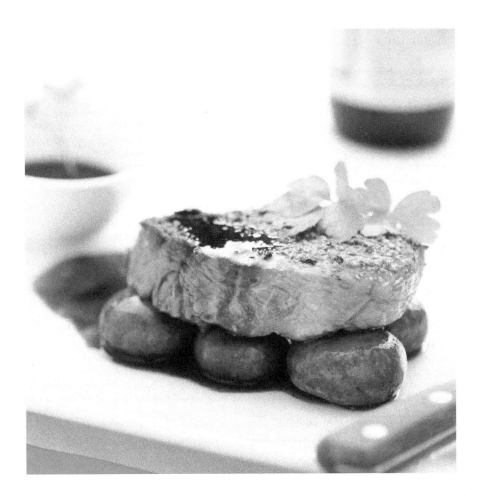

Lemony Mustard Pork Roast

Preparation time: 10 minutes
Cooking time: 60 minutes
Servings: 5

Ingredients:
2 pounds (907 g) pork loin roast, trimmed
1½ tablespoons olive oil
1 tablespoon fresh lemon juice
1 tablespoon pork rub seasoning blend
1 tablespoon stone-ground mustard

Directions:
Pat the pork loin roast dry.
Massage the pork loin roast with the olive oil. Then, sprinkle the lemon juice, pork rub seasoning blend, and mustard over all sides of
the roast.
Prepare a grill for indirect heat. Grill the pork loin roast over indirect heat for about 1 hour. Let the grilled pork loin stand for 10 minutes before slicing and serving. Bon appétit!

Nutrition:
calories: 385 | fat: 20.2g | protein: 48.0g | carbs: 0.1g | net carbs: 0g | fiber: 0.1g

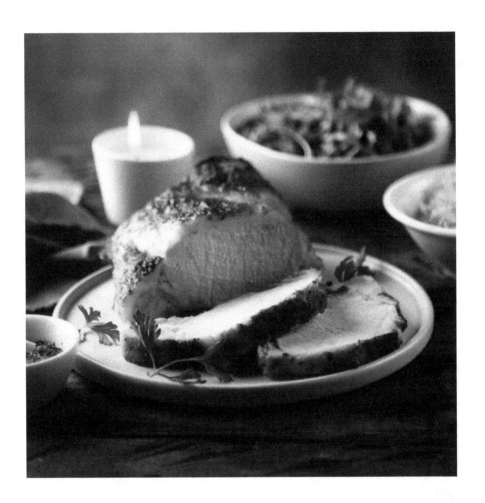

Roasted Pork Loin with Collard

Preparation time: 10 minutes
Cooking time: 60 minutes
Servings: 4

Ingredients:
2 tablespoons olive oil
Salt and black pepper, to taste
1½ pounds (680 g) pork loin
A pinch of dry mustard
1 teaspoon hot red pepper flakes
½ teaspoon ginger, minced
cup collard greens, chopped
garlic cloves, minced
½ lemon, sliced ¼ cup water

Directions:
In a bowl, combine the ginger with salt, mustard, and black pepper. Add in the meat, toss to coat. Heat the oil in a saucepan over medium heat, brown the pork on all sides, for 10 minutes.
Transfer to the oven and roast for 40 minutes at 390°F (199°C). To the saucepan, add collard greens, lemon slices, garlic, and water; cook for 10 minutes. Serve on a platter and sprinkle pan juices on top.

Nutrition:
calories: 431
fat: 23.0g
protein: 45.0g
carbs: 3.6g
net carbs: 3.0g
fiber: 0.6g

Rosemary Pork Chops with Kalamata Olives

Preparation time: 10 minutes
Cooking time: 40 minutes
Servings: 4

Ingredients:
4 pork chops, bone-in
Salt and ground black pepper, to taste
1 teaspoon dried rosemary
3 garlic cloves, peeled and minced
½ cup kalamata olives, pitted and sliced
2 tablespoons olive oil
¼ cup vegetable broth

Directions:
Season pork chops with black pepper and salt, and add in a roasting pan. Stir in the garlic, olives, olive oil, broth, and rosemary, set in the oven at 425°F (220°C), and bake for 10 minutes. Reduce heat to 350°F (180°C) and roast for 25 minutes. Slice the pork and sprinkle with pan juices all over to serve.

Nutrition:
calories: 416
fat: 25.1g
protein: 36.1g
carbs: 2.9g
net carbs: 2.1g
fiber: 0.8g

Beef and Lamb

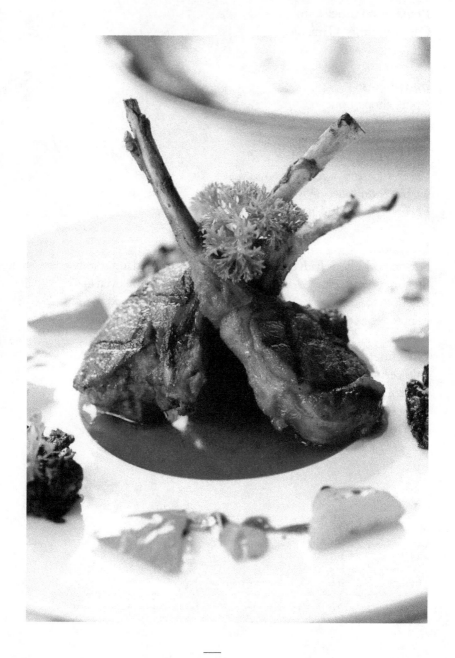

Thai Beef Steak with Mushrooms

Preparation time: 15 minutes
Cooking time: 25 minutes
Servings: 6

Ingredients:
1 cup beef stock
4 tablespoons butter
¼ teaspoon garlic powder ¼ teaspoon onion powder
1 tablespoon coconut aminos
1½ teaspoons lemon pepper
1 pound (454 g) beef steak, cut into strips
Salt and black pepper, to taste
1 cup shiitake mushrooms, sliced
3 green onions, chopped
1 tablespoon thai red curry paste

Directions:
Melt butter in a pan over medium heat, add in the beef, season with garlic powder, black pepper, salt, and onion powder and cook for 4 minutes. Mix in the mushrooms and stir-fry for 5 minutes.
Pour in the stock, coconut aminos, lemon pepper, and thai curry paste and cook for 15 minutes. Serve sprinkled with the green onions.

Nutrition:
calories: 225
fat: 15.1g
protein: 18.9g
carbs: 4.1g
net carbs: 2.9g
fiber: 1.2g

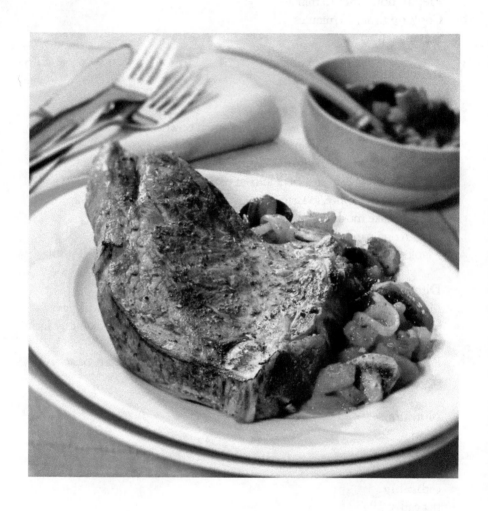

Beef and Pimiento in Zucchini Boats

Preparation time: 10 minutes
Cooking time: 25 minutes
Servings: 4

Ingredients:
4 zucchinis
2 tablespoons olive oil
1½ pounds (680 g) ground beef
medium red onion, chopped
tablespoons chopped pimiento
Pink salt and black pepper to taste
1 cup grated yellow Cheddar cheese

Directions:
Preheat oven to 350°F (180°C).
Lay the zucchinis on a flat surface, trim off the ends and cut in half lengthwise. Scoop out the pulp from each half with a spoon to make shells. Chop the pulp. Heat oil in a skillet; add the ground beef, red onion, pimiento, and zucchini pulp, and season with salt and black pepper. Cook for 6 minutes while stirring to break up lumps until beef is no longer pink. Turn the heat off. Spoon the beef into the boats and sprinkle with Cheddar cheese.
Place on a greased baking sheet and cook to melt the cheese for 15 minutes until zucchini boats are tender. Take out, cool for 2 minutes, and serve warm with a mixed green salad.

Nutrition:
calories: 334
fat: 24.0g
protein: 17.9g
carbs: 7.6g
net carbs: 6.9g
fiber: 0.7g

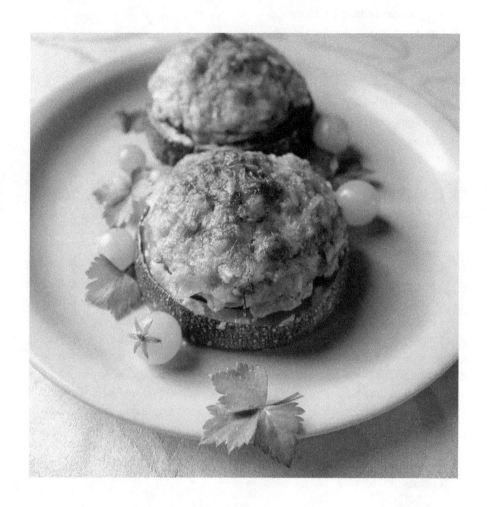

Lemony Beef Rib Roast

Preparation time: 15 minutes
Cooking time: 35 minutes
Servigs: 6

Ingredients:
5 pounds (2.3 kg) beef rib roast, on the bone
3 heads garlic, cut in half
3 tablespoons olive oil
6 shallots, peeled and halved
lemons, zested and juiced
tablespoons mustard seeds
3 tablespoons Swerve
Salt and black pepper to taste
3 tablespoons thyme leaves

Directions:
Preheat oven to 450°F (235°C). Place garlic heads and shallots in a roasting dish, toss with olive oil, and bake for 15 minutes. Pour lemon juice on them. Score shallow crisscrosses patterns on the meat and set aside.
Mix Swerve, mustard seeds, thyme, salt, pepper, and lemon zest to make a rub; and apply it all over the beef. Place the beef on the shallots and garlic; cook in the oven for 15 minutes. Reduce the heat to 400°F (205°C), cover the dish with foil, and continue cooking for 5 minutes.
Once ready, remove the dish, and let sit covered for 15 minutes before slicing.

Nutrition:
calories: 555
fat: 38.5g
protein: 58.3g
carbs: 7.7g
net carbs: 2.4g
fiber: 5.3g

Easy Balsamic Beef Chuck Roast

Preparation time: 15 minutes
Cooking: time: 7 to 8 hours
Servings: 8

Ingredients:
3 tablespoons of extra-virgin olive oil, divided
2 pounds (907 g) boneless beef chuck roast
1 cup beef broth
½ cup balsamic vinegar
1 tablespoon minced garlic
1 tablespoon granulated erythritol
½ teaspoon red pepper flakes
1 tablespoon chopped fresh thyme

Directions:
Lightly grease the insert of the slow cooker with 1 tablespoon of the olive oil.
In a large skillet over medium-high heat, heat the remaining 2 tablespoons of the olive oil. Add the beef and brown on all sides, about 7 minutes total.
Transfer to the insert.
In a small bowl, whisk together the broth, balsamic vinegar, garlic, erythritol, red pepper flakes, and thyme until blended.
Pour the sauce over the beef.
Cover and cook on low for 7 to 8 hours.
Serve warm.

Nutrition:
calories: 477
fat: 39.0g
protein: 27.8g
carbs: 1.1g
net carbs: 1.1g
fiber: 0g

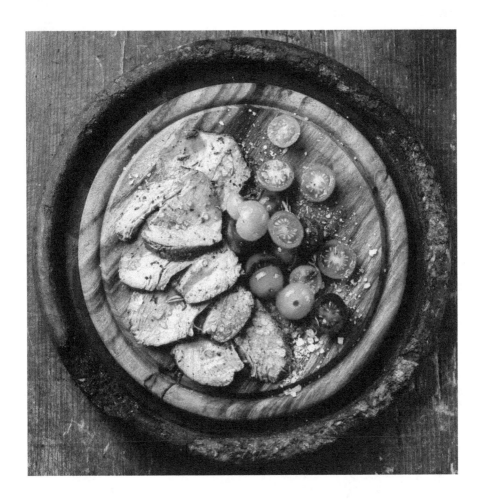

Braised Beef Short Ribs with Sweet Onion

Preparation time: 10 minutes
Cooking time: 7 to 8 hours
Servings: 8

Ingredients:
tablespoon extra-virgin olive oil
pounds (907 g) beef short ribs
sweet onion, sliced
cups beef broth
2 tablespoons granulated erythritol
2 tablespoons balsamic vinegar
2 teaspoons dried thyme
1 teaspoon hot sauce

Directions:
Lightly grease the insert of the slow cooker with the olive oil.
Place the ribs, onion, broth, erythritol, balsamic vinegar, thyme, and hot sauce in the insert.
Cover and cook on low for 7 to 8 hours.
Serve warm.

Nutrition:
calories: 475
fat: 42.8g
protein: 17.9g
carbs: 2.0g
net carbs: 2.0g
fiber: 0g

Herbed Veggie and Beef Stew

Preparation time: 10 minutes
Cooking time: 25 minutes
Serves 4

Ingredients:
pound (454 g)ground beef
tablespoons olive oil
onion, chopped
garlic cloves, minced
14 ounces (397 g) canned diced tomatoes
1 tablespoon dried rosemary
1 tablespoon dried sage
1 tablespoon dried oregano
1 tablespoon dried basil
tablespoon dried marjoram
Salt and black pepper, to taste
carrots, sliced
2 celery stalks, chopped
1 cup vegetable broth

Directions:
Set a pan over medium heat, add in the olive oil, onion, celery, and garlic, and sauté for 5 minutes. Place in the beef, and cook for 6 minutes. Stir in the tomatoes, carrots, broth, black pepper, oregano, marjoram, basil, rosemary, salt, and sage, and simmer for 15 minutes. Serve and enjoy!

Nutrition:
calories: 254
fat: 13.1g
protein: 29.9g
carbs: 10.1g
net carbs: 5.1g
fiber: 5.0g

Fish and Seafood

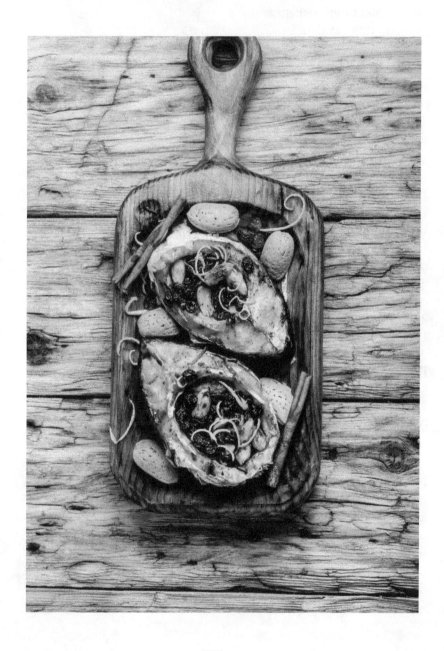

Coconut Catfish

Preparation time: 10 minutes
Cooking time: 2.5 hours
Servings: 3

Ingredients:
3 catfish fillets
1 teaspoon coconut shred
½ cup of coconut milk
teaspoon sesame seeds
tablespoons fish sauce
cup of water
tablespoons soy sauce

Directions:
Pour water in the slow cooker.
Add soy sauce, fish sauce, sesame seeds, and coconut milk.
Then add coconut shred and catfish fillets.
Cook the fish on high for 2.5 hours.

Nutrition:
329 calories,
27.3g protein,
3.9g carbohydrates,
22.7g fat,
1.2g fiber,
75mg cholesterol,
1621mg sodium,
682mg potassium.

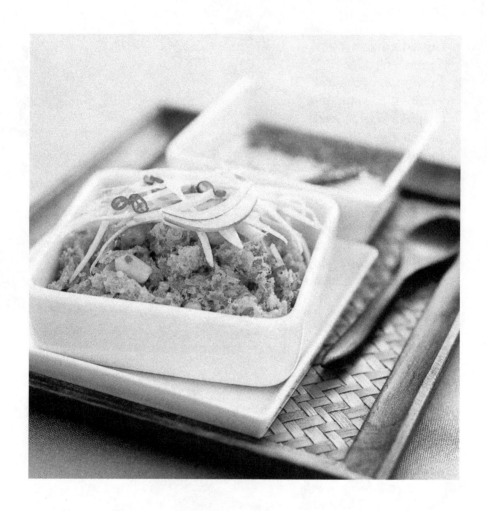

Tuna Casserole

Preparation time: 15 minutes
Cooking time: 6 hours
Servings: 4

Ingredients:
 1 cup mushrooms, sliced
½ cup corn kernels, frozen
8 oz tuna, chopped
1 teaspoon Italian seasonings
1 cup chicken stock
½ cup Cheddar cheese, shredded
1 tablespoon sesame oil

Directions:
Heat the sesame oil in the skillet.
Add mushrooms and roast them for 5 minutes on medium heat.
Then transfer the mushrooms in the slow cooker and flatten in one layer.
After this, mix Italian seasonings with tuna and put over the mushrooms.
Then top the fish with corn kernels and cheese.
Add chicken stock.
Cook the casserole on Low for 7 hours.

Nutrition:
219 calories,
19.9g protein,
4.7g carbohydrates,
13.4g fat,
0.7g fiber,
33mg cholesterol,
311mg sodium,
315mg potassium.

Salmon and Cucumber Panzanella

Preparation time: 15 minutes
Cooking time: 10 minutes
Servings: 4

Ingredients:
1 pound (454 g) skinned salmon, cut into 4 steaks each
1 cucumber, peeled, seeded, cubed
Salt and black pepper to taste
8 black olives, pitted and chopped
tablespoon capers, rinsed
large tomatoes, diced
tablespoons red wine vinegar
¼ cup thinly sliced red onion
3 tablespoons olive oil
2 slices zero carb bread, cubed
¼ cup thinly sliced basil leaves

Directions:
Preheat a grill to 350°F (180°C) and prepare the salad. In a bowl, mix the cucumbers, olives, pepper, capers, tomatoes, wine vinegar, onion, olive oil, bread, and basil leaves. Let sit for the flavors to incorporate.
Season the salmon steaks with salt and pepper; grill them on both sides for 8 minutes in total. Serve the salmon steaks warm on a bed of the veggies' salad.

Nutrition:
calories: 339
fat: 21.6g
protein: 28.6g
carbs: 5.3g
net carbs: 3.2g
fiber: 2.1g

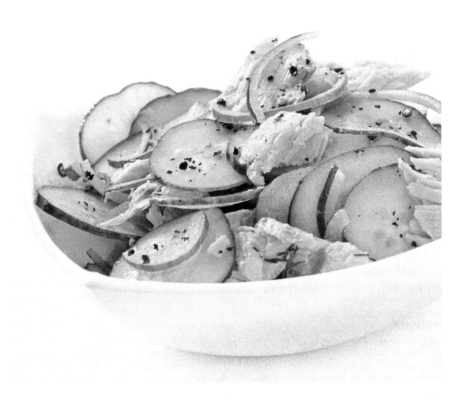

Cioppino

Preparation Time: 15 minutes
Cooking Time: 30 minutes
Servings: 6

Ingredients:
2 tablespoons olive oil
1/2 onion, chopped
2 celery stalks, sliced
1 red bell pepper, chopped
tablespoon minced garlic
cups fish stock
1 (15-ounce) can coconut milk
cup crushed tomatoes
tablespoons tomato paste
tablespoon chopped fresh basil
teaspoons chopped fresh oregano
1/2 teaspoon of sea salt
1/2 teaspoon freshly ground black pepper
1/4 teaspoon red pepper flakes
10 ounces salmon, cut into 1-inch pieces
1/2 pound shrimp, peeled and deveined
12 clams or mussels, cleaned and debearded but in the shell

Directions:
Sauté the vegetables. In a pot, warm the olive oil. Add the onion, celery, red bell pepper, and garlic and sauté until they've softened about 4 minutes. Make the soup base. Stir in the fish stock, coconut milk, crushed tomatoes, tomato paste, basil, oregano, salt, pepper, and red pepper flakes. Boil then simmer the soup for 10 minutes. Add the seafood. Stir in the salmon and simmer until it goes opaque about 5 minutes. Add the shrimp and simmer until they're almost cooked through about 3 minutes. Add the mussels. Serve.

Nutrition:
Calories: 321; Fat: 11.1g; Fiber: 16g; Carbohydrates:4.2 g; Protein: 16.4g

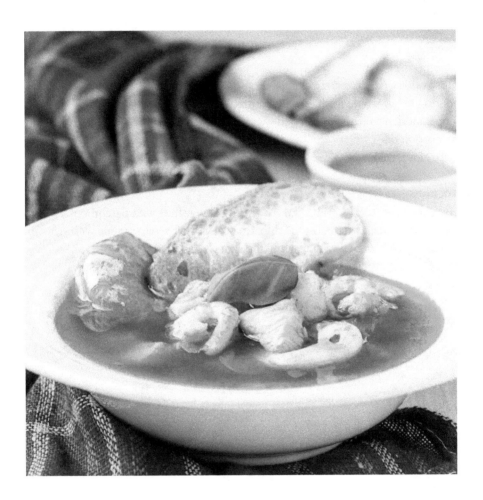

Sardines with Zoodles

Preparation time: 10 minutes
Cooking time: 15 minutes
Servings: 4

Ingredients:
2 tablespoons olive oil
4 cups zoodles (spiralized zucchini)
1 pound (454 g) whole fresh sardines, gutted and cleaned
½ cup sundried tomatoes, chopped
1 tablespoon dill
1 garlic clove, minced

Directions:
Preheat the oven to 350°F (180°C) and line a baking sheet with parchment paper. Arrange the sardines on the dish, drizzle with olive oil, sprinkle with salt and pepper. Bake for 10 minutes until the skin is crispy.
Warm oil in a skillet and stir-fry zucchini, garlic and tomatoes for 5 minutes.
Transfer the sardines to a plate and serve with the veggie pasta.

Nutrition:
calories: 432
fat: 28.2g
protein: 32.3g
carbs: 7.1g
net carbs: 5.4g
fiber: 1.7g

Dijon-Tarragon Salmon

Preparation time: 10 minutes
Cooking time: 10 minutes
Servings: 4

Ingredients:
4 salmon fillets
¾ teaspoon fresh thyme
tablespoon butter
¾ teaspoon tarragon Salt and black pepper to taste
Sauce:
¼ cup Dijon mustard
tablespoons white wine
½ teaspoon tarragon
¼ cup heavy cream

Directions:
Season the salmon with thyme, tarragon, salt, and black pepper. Melt the butter in a pan over medium heat. Add salmon and cook for about 4-5 minutes on both sides until the salmon is cooked through. Remove to a warm dish and cover.
To the same pan, add the sauce ingredients over low heat and simmer until the sauce is slightly thickened, stirring continually. Cook for 60 seconds to infuse the flavors and adjust the seasoning. Serve the salmon, topped with the sauce.

Nutrition:
calories: 538
fat: 26.5g
protein: 66.9g
carbs: 2.1g
net carbs: 1.4g
fiber: 0.7g

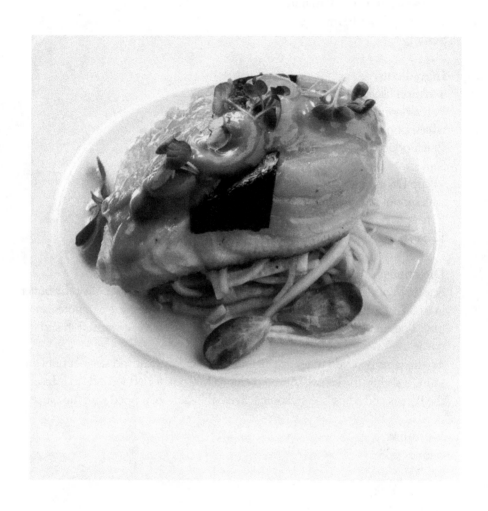

Soups

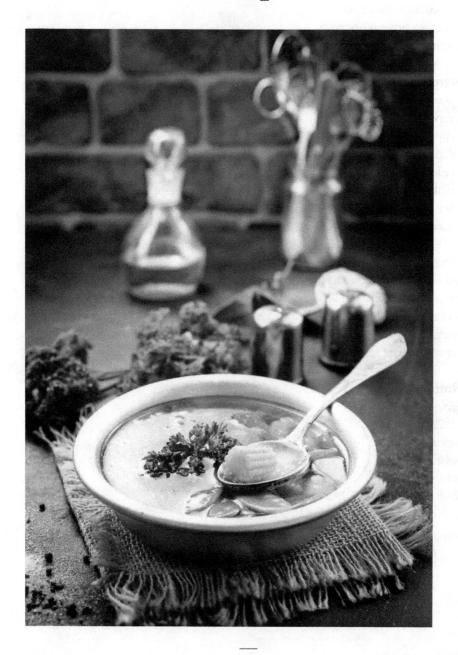

Turkey Taco Soup

Preparation time: 10 minutes
Cooking time: 4 hours
Servings: 6

Ingredients:
1 pound (454 g) ground turkey
5 cups chicken bone broth (you can also use regular chicken broth)
1 cup canned diced tomatoes (no sugar added)
1 cup whipped cream cheese
1 yellow onion, chopped
1 tablespoon chili powder
1 teaspoon cumin
1 teaspoon garlic powder 1 teaspoon onion powder

Directions:
Add all the ingredients to the base of a Crock-Pot minus the cream cheese and cover with the chicken broth.
Set on high and cook for 4 hours adding in the cream cheese at the 3.5 hour mark.
Stir well before serving.

Nutrition:
calories: 336
fat: 22.9g
protein: 27.9g
carbs: 5.9g
net carbs: 4.8g
fiber: 1.1g

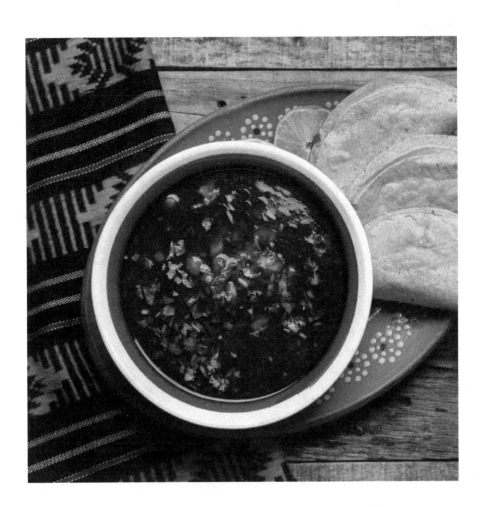

Spiced Lasagna Soup

Preparation time: 10 minutes
Cooking time: 4 hours
Servings: 2

Ingredients:
2 sheets of lasagna noodles, crushed
1 oz. Parmesan, grated
1 teaspoon ground turmeric
yellow onion, diced
cups ground beef
6 cups beef broth
½ cup tomatoes, chopped
1 tablespoon dried basil

Directions:
Roast the ground beef in the hot skillet for 4 minutes. Stir it constantly and transfer in the slow cooker.
Add turmeric, onion, and tomatoes, basil, and beef broth.
Stir the soup, add lasagna noodles, and close the lid.
Cook the soup on High for 6 hours.
Top the cooked soup with Parmesan.

Nutrition:
208 calories,
17.8g protein,
14.6g carbohydrates,
8.3g fat,
0.7g fiber,
40mg cholesterol,
840mg sodium,
390mg potassium.

Chicken Garlic Soup

Preparation time: 10 minutes
Cooking time: 15 minutes
Servings: 6

Ingredients:
2 boneless, skinless chicken breasts
4 cups chicken broth
½ cup whipped cream cheese
3 cloves garlic, chopped
1 teaspoon thyme
1 teaspoon salt
¼ teaspoon black pepper
1 tablespoon butter

Directions:
Preheat a stockpot over medium heat with the butter.
Add the chicken and brown until completely cooked through. Remove from heat.
Shred the chicken and add it back to the stockpot along with the remaining ingredients minus the cream cheese.
Bring to a simmer.
Add in the cream cheese and whisk until there are no more clumps.
Simmer for 10 minutes and serve.

Nutrition:
calories: 130
fat: 6.1g
protein: 15.9g
carbs: 2.1g
net carbs: 2.1g
fiber: 0g

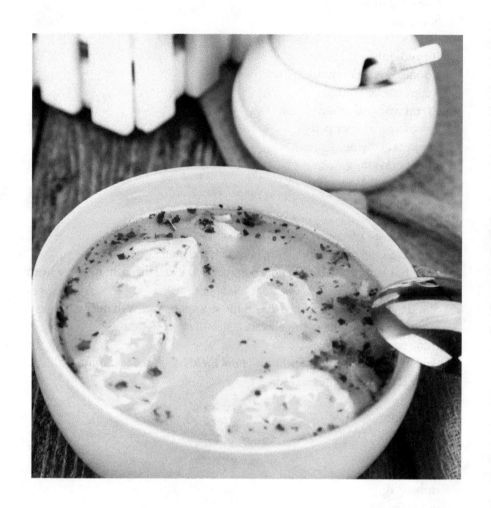

Beef and Mushroom Soup

Preparation time: 10 minutes
Cooking time: 40 minutes
Servings: 6

Ingredients:
1 pound (454 g) beef chuck, cubed
1½ cups cremini mushrooms
6 cups beef broth
½ cup heavy cream
½ cup whipped cream cheese
yellow onion, chopped
cloves garlic, chopped
Salt and pepper, to taste
1 tablespoon coconut oil, for cooking

Directions:
Add the coconut oil to a skillet and brown the beef.
Once cooked, add the beef to the base of a stockpot with all of the ingredients minus the heavy cream. Mix well.
Bring to a simmer and whisk again until the cream cheese is mixed evenly into the soup.
Cook for 30 minutes.
Warm the heavy cream, and then add to the soup.

Nutrition:
calories: 316
fat: 18.9g
protein: 30.1g
carbs: 5.0g
net carbs: 4.0g
fiber: 1.0g

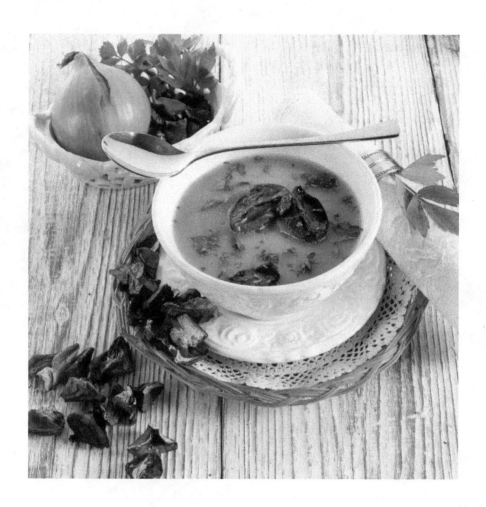

Pork Soup

Preparation time: 10 minutes
Cooking time: 25 minutes
Servings: 5

Ingredients:
2 teaspoons olive oil
pound (454 g)ground pork
shallots, chopped
1 celery stalk, chopped
1 fresh Italian pepper, deveined and chopped
5 cups beef bone broth
2 tablespoons fresh cilantro, roughly chopped

Directions:
Heat 1 teaspoon of the olive oil in a soup pot over a medium-high flame.
Brown the ground pork until no longer pink or about 4 minutes, crumbling with a spatula; reserve.
In the same pot, heat the remaining teaspoon of olive oil. Sauté the shallot until just tender and fragrant.
Add in the chopped celery and Italian pepper along with the reserved cooked pork.
Pour in the beef bone broth. When it comes to a boil, turn the heat to simmer. Let it simmer, partially covered, for 25 minutes until everything is cooked through.
Season with salt to taste, ladle into soup bowls, and garnish each serving with fresh cilantro. Bon appétit!

Nutrition:
calories: 293
fat: 20.5g
protein: 23.5g
carbs: 1.5g
net carbs: 1.3g
fiber: 0.2g

Beef, Tomato, and Zucchini Soup

Preparation time: 20 minutes
Cooking time: 6 hours
Servings: 6

Ingredients:
3 tablespoons extra-virgin olive oil, divided
pound (454 g) ground beef
½ sweet onion, chopped
teaspoons minced garlic
4 cups beef broth
1 (28-ounce / 794-g) can diced tomatoes, undrained
zucchini, diced
1½ tablespoons dried basil
teaspoons dried oregano
4 ounces (113 g) cream cheese
1 cup shredded Mozzarella

Directions:
Lightly grease the insert of the slow cooker with 1 tablespoon of the olive oil.
In a large skillet over medium-high heat, heat the remaining 2 tablespoons of the olive oil. Add the ground beef and sauté until it is cooked through, about 6 minutes.
Add the onion and garlic and sauté for an additional 3 minutes.
Transfer the meat mixture to the insert.
Stir in the broth, tomatoes, zucchini, basil, and oregano.
Cover and cook on low for 6 hours.
Stir in the cream cheese and Mozzarella and serve.

Nutrition:
calories: 473 | fat: 36.1g | protein: 29.9g | carbs: 8.9g | net carbs: 6.0g | fiber: 2.9g

Snack and Appetizers

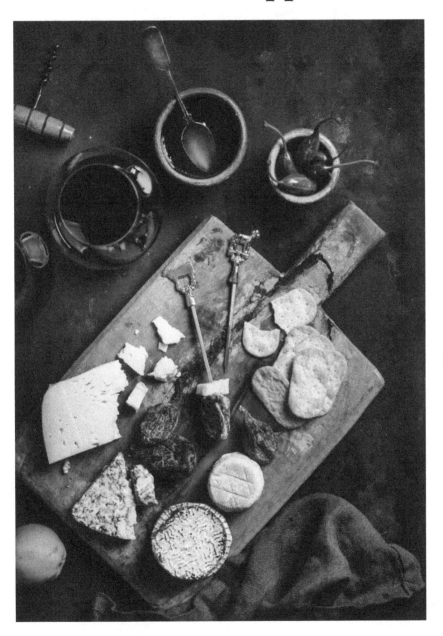

Pork Skewers with Greek Dipping Sauce

Preparation time: 15 minutes
Cooking time: 10 minutes
Servings: 2

Ingredients:
½ pound (227 g) pork loin, cut into bite-sized pieces
2 garlic cloves, pressed
1 scallion stalk, chopped
¼ cup dry red wine
1 thyme sprig
1 rosemary sprig
1 tablespoon lemon juice
1 teaspoon stone ground mustard
1 tablespoon olive oil
Dipping Sauce:
½ cup Greek yogurt
½ teaspoon dill, ground
½ Lebanese cucumber, grated
teaspoon garlic, minced
Sea salt, to taste
½ teaspoon ground black pepper
tablespoons cilantro leaves, roughly chopped

Directions:
Place the pork loin in a ceramic dish; add in the garlic, scallions, wine, thyme, rosemary, lemon juice, mustard, and olive oil. Let them marinate in your refrigerator for 2 to 3 hours Thread the pork pieces onto bamboo skewers. Grill them for 5 to 6 minutes per side. Meanwhile, whisk the remaining ingredients until well mixed. Serve the pork skewers with the sauce for dipping and enjoy!

Nutrition:
calories: 313 | fat: 20.0g | protein: 29.2g | carbs: 2.2g | net carbs: 1.6g | fiber: 0.6g

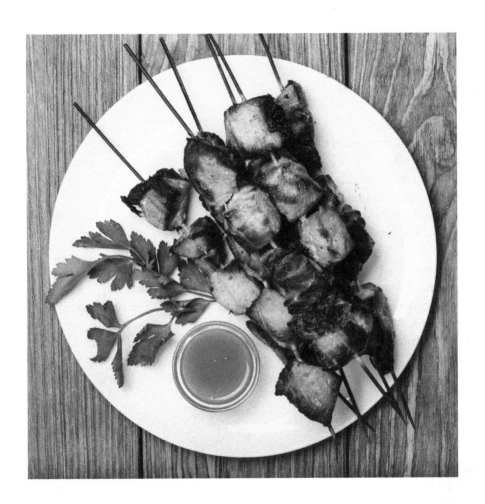

Caribbean Baked Wings

Preparation time: 15 minutes
Cooking time: 45 minutes
Servings: 2

Ingredients:
4 chicken wings
tablespoon coconut aminos
tablespoons rum
2 tablespoons butter
tablespoon onion powder1 tablespoon garlic powder
½ teaspoon salt
¼ teaspoon freshly ground black pepper
½ teaspoon red pepper flakes
¼ teaspoon dried dill
tablespoons sesame seeds

Directions:
Pat dry the chicken wings. Toss the chicken wings with the remaining ingredients until well coated. Arrange the chicken wings on a parchment-lined baking sheet.
Bake in the preheated oven at 420°F (216°C) for 45 minutes until golden brown.
Serve with your favorite sauce for dipping. Bon appétit!

Nutrition:
calories: 287
fat: 18.6g
protein: 15.5g
carbs: 5.1g
net carbs: 3.3g
fiber: 1.8g

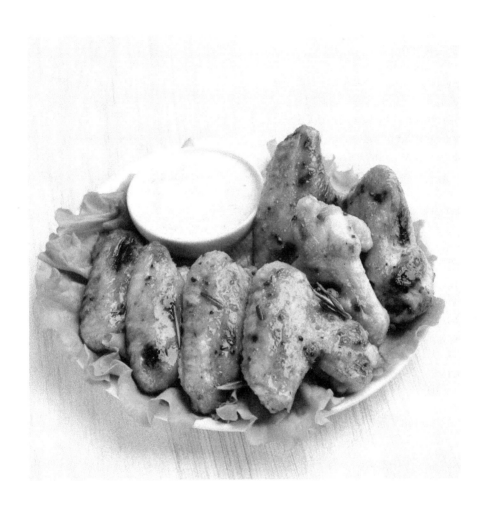

BBQ Chicken Dip

Preparation time: 10 minutes
Cooking time: 1 hour and 30 minutes
Servings: 10

Ingredients:
and ½ cups bob sauce
1 small red onion, chopped
24 ounces cream cheese, cubed
cups rotisserie chicken, shredded
bacon slices, cooked and crumbled
1 plum tomato, chopped
½ cup cheddar cheese, shredded 1 tablespoon green onions, chopped

Directions:
In your slow cooker, mix bob sauce with onion, cream cheese, rotisserie chicken, bacon, tomato, cheddar and green onions, stir, cover and cook on Low for 1 hour and 30 minutes.
Divide into bowls and serve.

Nutrition
Calories 251,
Fat 4,
Fiber 6,
Carbs 10,
Protein 4

Sweet Onion Dip

Preparation Time: 15 minutes
Cooking Time: 25-30 minutes
Servings: 4

Ingredients:
3 cup sweet onion chopped
tsp. pepper sauce
cups Swiss cheese shredded
Ground black pepper
2 cups mayonnaise   1/4 cup horseradish

Directions:
Take a bowl, add sweet onion, horseradish, pepper sauce, mayonnaise, and
Swiss cheese, mix them well and transfer into the pie plate.
Preheat oven at 375.
Now put the plate into the oven and bake for 25 to 30 minutes until edges turn
golden brown.
Sprinkle pepper to taste and serve with crackers.

Nutrition:
Calories: 278
Fat: 11.4g
Fiber: 4.1g
Carbohydrates:2.9 g
Protein: 6.9g

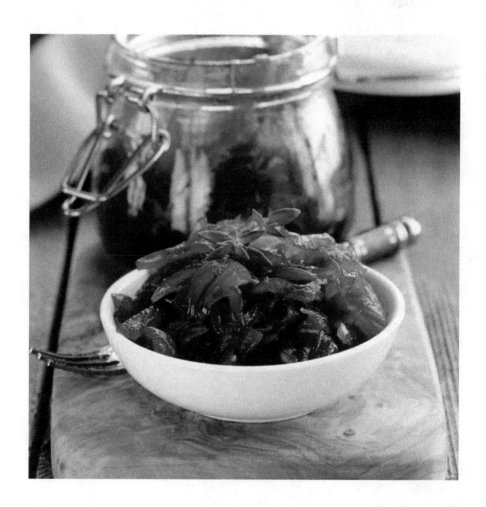

Sardine Pepper Boats

Preparation time: 10 minutes
Cooking time: 10 minutes
Servings: 3

Ingredients:
2 eggs
½ red onion, chopped
½ teaspoon garlic clove, minced
ounces (57 g) canned boneless sardines, drained and chopped
¼ freshly ground black pepper
½ cup tomatoes, chopped
¼ cup mayonnaise
tablespoons Ricotta cheese
3 bell peppers, deveined and halved

Directions:
Place the eggs and water in a saucepan; bring to a rapid boil; immediately remove from the heat.
Allow it to sit, covered, for 10 minutes. Then, discard the shells, rinse the eggs under cold water, and chop them.
Thoroughly combine the onion, garlic, sardines, black pepper, tomatoes, mayonnaise, and cheese.
Stuff the pepper halves and serve well chilled. Bon appétit!
ù
Nutrition:
calories: 372
fat: 31.2g
protein: 16.1g
carbs: 5.9g
net carbs: 4.5g
fiber: 1.4g

Jalapeño Poppers

Preparation time: 30 minutes
Cooking time: 4 hours
Servings: 24

Ingredients:
24 slices bacon
1 (8-ounce) package cream cheese, at room temperature
¼ cup sour cream
¼ cup grated Cheddar cheese
12 jalapeños, seeded and halved lengthwise
⅓ Cup Chicken Stock (or store-bought) or water

Directions:
Place the bacon in a large skillet over medium heat and cook, turning frequently, until partially cooked but still bendable. Drain the bacon on paper towels and let cool. In a medium bowl, mix together the cream cheese, sour cream, and Cheddar cheese until well blended. .Divide the cheese mixture evenly among the jalapeño halves. Wrap each stuffed jalapeño half with a slice of bacon; secure the bacon with a toothpick. .Pour the chicken stock into a 3-to 4-quart slow cooker and add the stuffed jalapeños. Cover and cook on low for 4 hours or on high for 2 hours. Using a slotted spoon, remove the stuffed jalapeños from the slow cooker. Serve hot or at room temperature.

Nutrition:
Calories: 89;
Fat: 7g;
Saturated Fat: 4g;
Cholesterol: 23mg;
Carbohydrates: 1g;
Fiber: <1g;
Protein: 5g;
Sodium: 205mg

Dessert

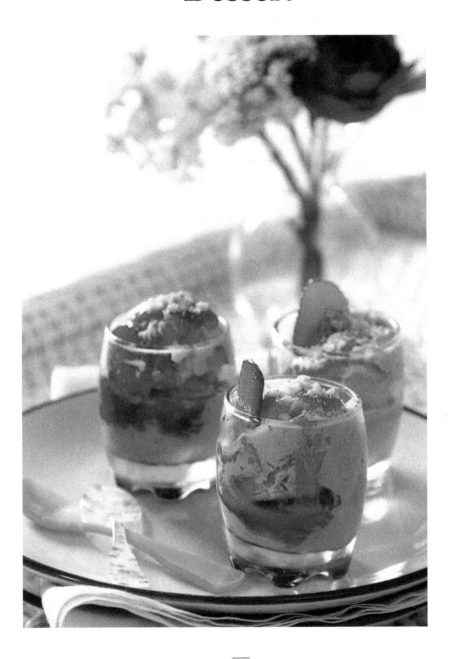

Lemon Almond Coconut Cake

Preparation Time: 20 minutes
Cooking Time: 40-45 minutes
Servings: 8

Ingredients:
250g almond
60g desiccated coconut
Pinch of salt
150g natural sugar 1 teaspoon vanilla extract zest of 1 large lemon
3 eggs
200g butter, melted
A handful of almond flakes

Directions:
Preheat oven to 180°C.
In a medium bowl, take almond, coconut, salt, sugar, vanilla, and lemon zest.
Mix in remaining ingredients.
Pour in a cake pan. Scatter with almond flakes.
Bake for approximately 40-45 minutes until lightly browned and cooked through the middle.

Nutrition:
Calories: 314
Fat: 12.4g
Fiber: 6.1g
Carbohydrates:3.1 g
Protein: 3.9g

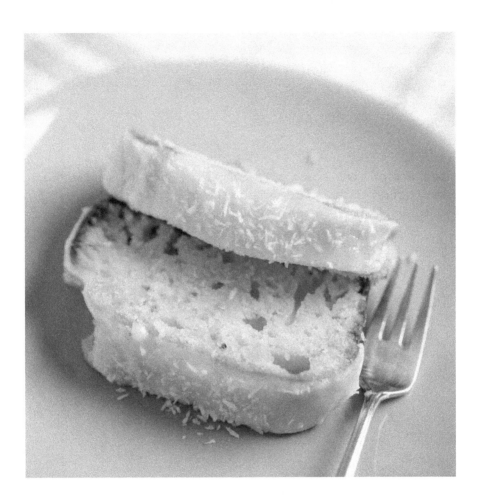

Coconut Jam

Preparation time: 10 minutes
Cooking time: 3 hours
Servings: 2

Ingredients:
½ cup coconut flesh, shredded
cup coconut cream
½ cup heavy cream
3 tablespoons sugar 1 tablespoon lemon juice

Directions:
In your slow cooker, mix the coconut cream with the lemon juice and the other ingredients, whisk, put the lid on and cook on Low for 3 hours.
Whisk well, divide into bowls and serve cold.

Nutrition
Calories 50,
Fat 1,
Fiber 1,
Carbs 10,

Berries Salad

Preparation time: 10 minutes
Cooking time: 1 hour
Servings: 2

Ingredients:
2 tablespoons brown sugar
1 tablespoon lime juice
1 tablespoon lime zest, grated
1 cup blueberries
½ cup cranberries
1 cup blackberries
1 cup strawberries
½ cup heavy cream

Directions:
In your slow cooker, mix the berries with the sugar and the other ingredients, toss, put the lid on and cook on High for 1 hour.
Divide the mix into bowls and serve.

Nutrition:
Calories 262,
Fat 7,
Fiber 2,
Carbs 5,
Protein 8

Almond Fudge Bars

Preparation time: 10 minutes
Cooking time: 0 minutes
Servings: 7

Ingredients:
1 cup almonds
4 tablespoons coconut flakes
4 tablespoons cacao powder, no sugar added
3 tablespoons coconut oil ¼ cup monk fruit powder

Directions:
Process all ingredients in your blender until everything is well combined, scraping down the sides as needed.
Press firmly into a parchment lined rectangular pan.
Cut into squares and serve your bars well chilled. Bon appétit!

Nutrition:
calories: 80
fat: 6.9g
protein: 0.6g
carbs: 4.6g
net carbs: 3.5g
fiber: 1.1g

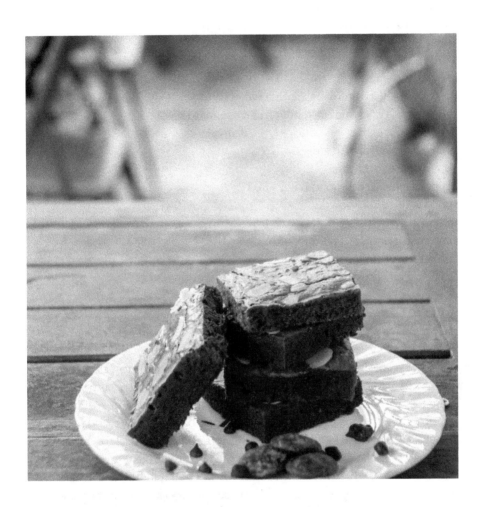

Simple Butter Cookies

Preparation time: 10 minutes
Cooking time: 20 minutes
Makes: 24

Ingredients:

1 cup granulated erythritol–monk fruit blend
8 tablespoons (1 stick) unsalted butter, at room temperature
teaspoon vanilla extract
large eggs, at room temperature
½ cup full-fat sour cream
2½ cups finely milled almond flour, sifted
1½ teaspoons baking powder
¼ teaspoon sea salt
1¼ cups confectioners' erythritol–monk fruit blend
½ cup full-fat sour cream
½ teaspoon vanilla extract

Direction:

Preheat the oven to 350°F (180°C). Line the baking sheet with parchment paper and set aside. In the medium bowl, using an electric mixer on high, combine the granulated erythritol–monk fruit blend, butter, and vanilla for 1 to 2 minutes, until light and fluffy, stopping and scraping the bowl once or twice, as needed. Add the eggs, one at a time, to the medium bowl, then add the sour cream. Mix until well incorporated. Next add the almond flour, baking powder, and salt and mix until just combined. Put the dough in the refrigerator and chill for 30 minutes. Drop the dough in tablespoons on the prepared baking sheet evenly spaced about 1 inch apart. Bake the cookies for 15 to 20 minutes, until lightly browned around the edges. Transfer the cookies to a cooling rack to fully cool, 15 to 20 minutes. In the small bowl, combine the confectioners' erythritol–monk fruit blend, sour cream, and vanilla. Once the cookies are fully cooled, using a spoon or pastry bag, drizzle the icing on top to serve. Store leftovers in the refrigerator for up to 5 days or freeze for up to 3 weeks.

Nutrition:

(2 Cookies) calories: 235 | fat: 21.9g | protein: 6.0g | carbs: 6.0g | net carbs: 4.0g | fiber: 2.0g

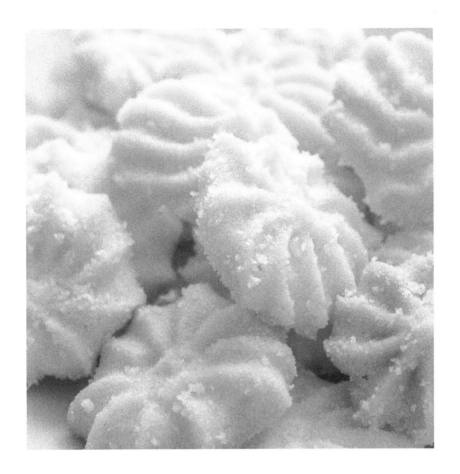

Lime and Coconut Panna Cotta

Preparation time: 10 minutes
Cooking time: 10 minutes
Servings: 4

Ingredients:
Coconut oil, for greasing
tablespoons unflavored gelatin
tablespoons cold water
1 (13.5-ounce / 383-g) can full-fat coconut milk
⅓ cup granulated erythritol–monk fruit blend; less sweet: 3 tablespoons
1 teaspoon grated lime zest
1 tablespoon freshly squeezed lime juice
½ teaspoon vanilla extract
⅛ teaspoon salt

Directions:
Grease the molds with coconut oil and set aside.
In the small bowl, soften the gelatin powder in the cold water and set aside.
In the medium saucepan, heat the coconut milk over medium heat until boiling.
Reduce the heat and simmer for a couple of minutes, until the cream begins to
thicken. While stirring, add the erythritol– monk fruit blend, lime zest, lime
juice, vanilla, and salt. Continue to stir to combine all the ingredients. Remove
from the heat and add the dissolved gelatin. Stir until the gelatin is dissolved.
Pour the mixture into the prepared molds and allow them to cool at room
temperature for about 30 minutes. Cover with plastic wrap and put in the
refrigerator for at least 4 hours before unmolding. To remove the panna cotta
from the molds, dip the molds in a bowl of hot water to help loosen. Serve
cold. Store leftovers in an airtight container or covered with plastic wrap in the
refrigerator for up to 3 days.

Nutrition:
calories: 211 | fat: 21.0g | protein: 5.1g | carbs: 2.9g | net carbs: 2.9g | fiber: 0g

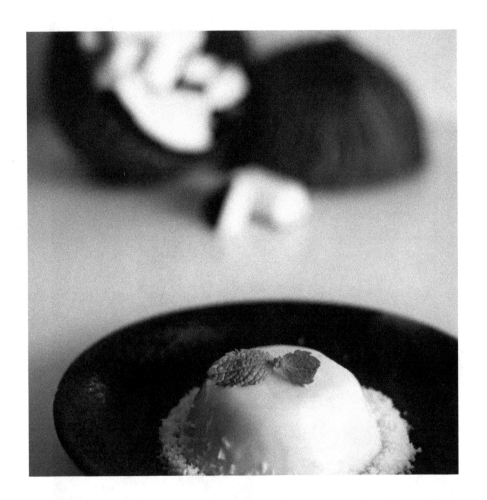

Drinks

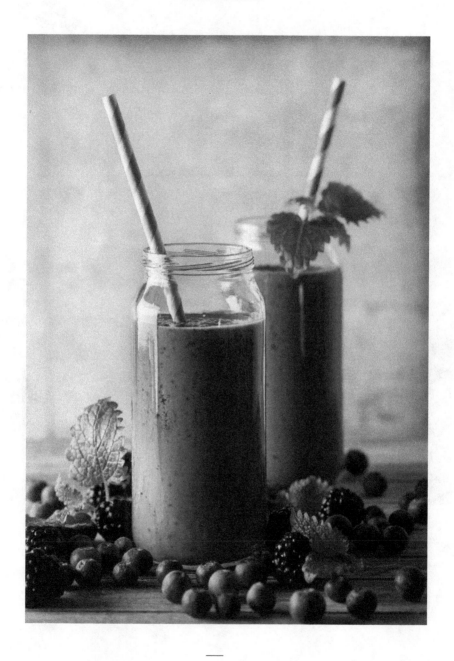

Blueberry Tofu Smoothie

Preparation Time: 15 minutes
Cooking Time: 0 minutes
Servings: 1

Ingredients:
6 ounces of silken tofu
1 medium banana
2/3 cups of soy milk
1 cup of frozen or fresh blueberries (divided)
1 tablespoon of honey 2-3 ice cubes (optional)

Directions:
Drain the silken tofu to remove the excess water (silken tofu as a high-water content)
Peele and slice the banana. Place the sliced banana on a baking sheet and freeze them. This process usually takes up to 15 minutes. This helps to make the smoothie thicker.
Get a blender. Blend the banana, tofu, and soy milk. This usually takes up to 30 seconds.
Add 1/2 cup of the blueberries to the banana, tofu, and soymilk. Then blend it until it is very smooth.
Put the remaining blueberries. Add honey and ice cubes. Blend it until it is well combined.
Serve and enjoy.

Nutrition:
Calories: 312
Fat: 9.5g
Fiber: 11.8g
Carbohydrates:2.7 g
Protein: 12.1g

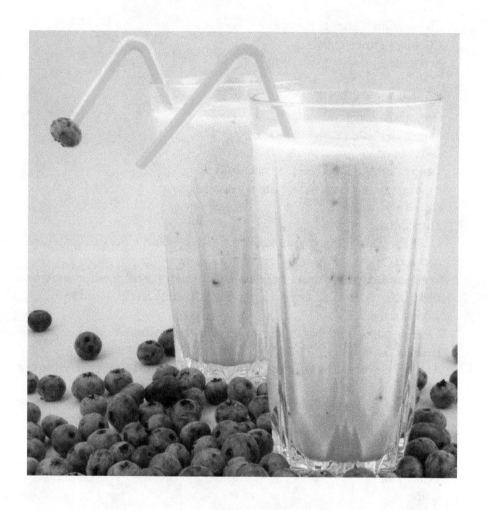

Raspberry Coulis

Preparation time: 3 minutes
Cooking time: 5 minutes
Makes: 1½ cups

Ingredients:
2 cups fresh or frozen red raspberries
2 tablespoons granulated erythritol
Combine the raspberries and sweetener in a small saucepan and cook over medium heat for 5 minutes, or until bubbling.
Blend with an immersion blender for 30 seconds or until liquefied, then pour the sauce through a fine-mesh strainer to remove any seed fragments. Let cool before using.
Store in an airtight container in the refrigerator for up to 1 week or in the freezer for up to 3 months.

Nutrition:
calories: 13
fat: 0g
protein: 0g
carbs: 2.6g
net carbs: 1.0g
fiber: 1.6g

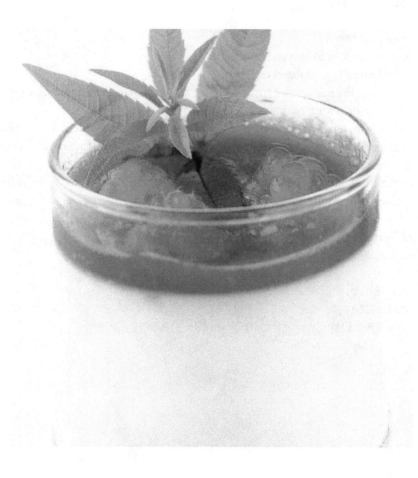

Marinara

Preparation time: 5 minutes
Cooking time: 0 minutes
Makes: 4 cups

Ingredients:
(28-ounce / 794-g) can peeled whole San Marzano tomatoes
¼ cup extra-virgin olive oil
tablespoons red wine vinegar
1 teaspoon dried basil leaves
1 teaspoon dried oregano leaves
1 teaspoon dried parsley leaves
1 teaspoon garlic powder 1 teaspoon kosher salt
1 teaspoon onion powder
½ teaspoon red pepper flakes
¼ teaspoon ground black pepper

Directions:
Place the tomatoes and olive oil in a blender and blend for 30 seconds, or until the desired consistency is reached. If you prefer a chunkier sauce, pulse instead of blending for about 15 seconds. Stir in
the remaining ingredients.
Store in an airtight container for up to 1 week in the refrigerator or 6 months in the freezer.

Nutrition:
calories: 85
fat: 6.8g
protein: 1.0g
carbs: 5.0g
net carbs: 3.0g
fiber: 2.0g

Ketchup

Preparation time: 5 minutes
Cooking time: 1 hour
Makes: 2 cups

Ingredients:
1 (28-ounce / 794-g) can tomato purée
⅓ cup granulated erythritol
¼ teaspoon cayenne pepper
½ cup white vinegar
1½ teaspoons dehydrated onions
½ teaspoon celery salt
½ teaspoon whole cloves
1 (1-inch) piece of cinnamon stick, broken

Directions:
Combine the tomato purée, sweetener, and cayenne pepper in a medium-sized saucepan and bring to a boil over medium heat, then reduce the heat to low. Simmer until it reduces by half, about 30 minutes, stirring occasionally.
Meanwhile, in another small saucepan, combine the vinegar, onions, celery salt, cloves, and cinnamon stick pieces. Bring to a boil, then remove from the heat. Strain out the solids.
Add the flavored vinegar to the tomato mixture. Simmer for another 20 minutes, or until the ketchup reaches the desired consistency. Remove from the heat and let cool.
Blend the cooled ketchup with an immersion blender or in a small blender until smooth. Store in a clean jar with an airtight lid for up to 1 month in the refrigerator.

Nutrition:
calories: 15
fat: 0g protein: 0g
carbs: 3.8g
net carbs: 2.8g
fiber: 1.0g

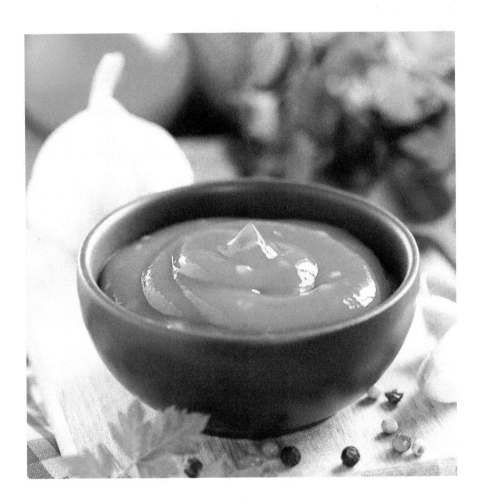

Creamy Duo-Cheese Dipping Sauce

Preparation time: 10 minutes
Cooking time: 0 minutes
Servings: 10

Ingredients:
4 ounces (113 g) Feta cheese
1 cup Asiago cheese, shredded
1 cup double cream
1 tablespoon paprika
Melt the cheese and cream in a saucepan over medium-low heat.
Transfer to a serving bowl and top with paprika.
Serve with fresh celery sticks if desired. Enjoy!

Nutrition:
calories: 127
fat: 10.8g
protein: 5.5g
carbs: 1.3g
net carbs: 1.3g
fiber: 0g

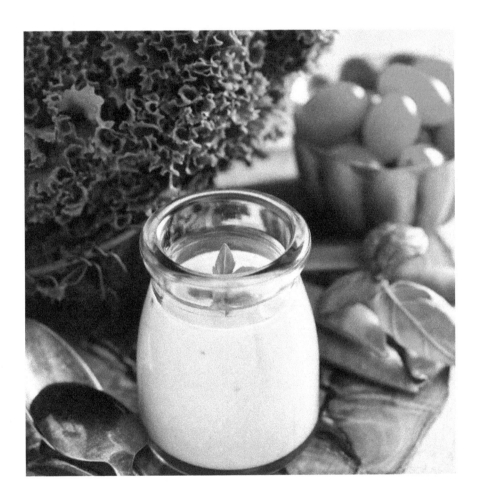

Remoulade

Preparation time: 5 minutes
Cooking time: 0 minutes
Makes: ½ cup

Ingredients:
⅓ cup sugar-free mayonnaise
1 tablespoon dill pickle relish
1 teaspoon Cajun Seasoning
1 teaspoon capers, drained
1 teaspoon Dijon mustard
1 teaspoon lemon juice
1 teaspoon prepared horseradish
½ teaspoon minced garlic

Directions:
Place all of the ingredients in a small bowl and mix well. Serve immediately or store in an airtight container in the refrigerator for up to 5 days.

Nutrition:
calories: 161
fat: 18.8g
protein: 0g
carbs: 1.1g
net carbs: 1.1g
fiber: 0g

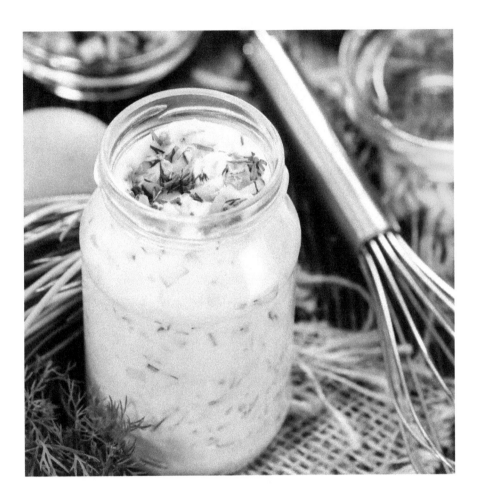

CPSIA information can be obtained
at www.ICGtesting.com
Printed in the USA
BVHW061037220321
603178BV00004B/221

9 781914 450228